BODYBUILDING
BARNEY STYLE

Jordan R. Bennefeld

CONTENTS

DEDICATION

This book is dedicated to anyone who puts forth the time and effort to better themselves. Not only is bodybuilding a physical exercise, but also mental. Stay true to yourself and your goals and NEVER let anyone tear you down.

CHAPTER 1

GET YOUR MIND RIGHT

Bodybuilding, where big is never big enough. Once you have fallen into its jaws, there is no getting out. You fall deeper and deeper into the pits, but you love every second of it. The sweat, the pain, the aching joints and sore muscles, we wouldn't trade it for the world. We love to torture ourselves to the point of perfection.

So what makes someone put themselves through it all? While it's nice to think that we do it to look more attractive for our partner, the reality is that we do it for ourselves. One might call that selfish, well I say, who gives a shit. My body is my vessel and I'll be damned if I don't strive to have the best damn vessel in the ocean. But while our ship may be the biggest, fastest, and strongest, it is nothing without a shrewd captain steering it.

Our minds our powerful, more powerful than we could ever imagine. I had heard people say this my whole life, but it wasn't until the Marine Corps that I understood what it meant. I was forced to push my body through excruciating tasks, tasks that I didn't think were possible. But you know what? I did it. I pushed my body past its limits and was successful. Anyone that has been in the military, played football, done martial arts, rock climbing, anything physical has experienced this. Once you shatter the doubt that you created in your own mind, you quickly realize that nothing is impossible.

I'm a strong believer in mind over matter. Now, that's not to say I'm going to bench 1,000 lbs just because I think I can, let's be realistic here. One of the things I tell people when lifting, is to "think big". It's somewhat difficult to put into words, but that's exactly what it is. Take your mind to the deepest of places and put all your heart into it. Imagine yourself as the Hulk, grip the bar as tight as you can, scream "I'm the Juggernaut bitch!" and lift that shit. You have to mentally visualize yourself as a massive, Icelandic freak of nature who just got his puppy stolen.

Anyone who is an avid gym-goer will tell you, if your mind isn't in the right place, it won't be enjoyable. That is where it gets tricky. You may have just broke up with Susie or maybe you wrecked your new Slowstang trying to do a burnout. Well, now you're pretty bummed out. You have to take all that frustration and funnel it to productivity.

Whether you're sad, angry, or just stressed out, you have to learn how to push all that to the back of your mind and focus on the task at hand. If you're unable to do it, you don't want it bad enough. Eric Thomas, a motivational speaker, is famous for the line "You have to want it as bad as you want to breathe." That statement couldn't be any more accurate. If you feel that sleeping or eating or taking it easy is more important than your goals, then don't bitch about it when you don't reach them. You have to tell yourself that this is your number one priority above anything else. Put your damn phone away, turn off the TV, tell your friends you're busy, and go out there and smash your goals.

Now, the funny part about being angry is...that shit it motivational. You go in there and make the weights your bitch. Be angry, be mad, and tear it up. As we all know, music helps you get into the zone as well. Personally, a little DMX, Em, and Manson will do the trick, but to each their own. If Tay Swizzle somehow pumps you up and you get the best work out of your life, then by all means, jam it out on max.

But back to the point at hand, our mind. You may have heard the term mind-muscle connection. I find that to help me out. You block everything out and focus everything you have on that particular muscle and that particular movement. A curl, for example, lift it slow and smooth and flex the entire time. Stare at it if you have to, but make sure that 100% of your attention is on that muscle. You will be surprised at the results as opposed to being on autopilot and just mindlessly lifting. The attention and focus that you give, staring at the girl in the squat rack, you need to give that to your muscles. Disregard everything else in the gym and have some damn bearing. Focus focus focus. I can't stress that enough.

Far too often we go to that autopilot mode and just go through the motions. We get complacent and do the same routine day after day. That will work if you just want to maintain, but why would you want to maintain? Who buys a car and says, "You know, this is enough horsepower for me." I know who says that, nobody. You have to break the cycle of going to the gym, doing the same lifts and lifting the same weight for 3 sets of 10. Those days are over, but we'll get into that later.

Something else that I can't stress enough is, listen to your body! Just because Tuesday is arm day, doesn't mean you feel like doing it every Tuesday. Maybe your shoulder hurts, so you would rather knock out some biceps and back. That is totally ok. While it is good to stick to a system or a schedule, you should always listen to your body. There have been times when I have done chest 3 times in one week just because it felt great. Other weeks I only did it once and killed my back instead. So again, stick to a system, but nothing so strict that you can't have a little wiggle room.

Plant the seed. Plant the seed in your head that this is what you want to do and this is your goal. Now water it. If you plant the seed in your mind that you want to achieve a certain goal, feed it so that it will grow. Before you know it, it will consume everything and that goal will turn into a reality. Remind yourself of it every day and surround yourself with things that contribute towards your goal. For those things that take you away from it, discard them. Get them out of your life, because fulfilling a commitment to yourself is hard, but it's even harder when you have things pulling you back.

CHAPTER 1.5

CAR-DAY-O

Cardio. I don't like it. I don't do too much of it, so this chapter will be short. If you want to burn some fat, do cardio I guess.

Ok, but on a real note, sometimes I will get on the stair stepper for about 15 mins after a workout. For the most part, I just take small breaks in between my sets in order to keep my heartrate up. Sometimes, about once a week or less, I'll do some burpees, flutter kicks, medicine ball exercises, and other calisthenic type exercises just to get a cardio/lean type of workout in. It feels good, but running and cardio in general just isn't my cup of tea.

CHAPTER 2

CHEST PECS TITS

This is the holy grail of muscle groups. Aside from traps, a solid chest is a true sign of strength and power. For some it comes easy, for others, not so much.

Growing up playing football, I have always strived to have a big chest. As we all know, defense wins games. So, I did everything I could to put on size. I would stay in the gym and work on my bench press day after day. With persistence and patience, it paid off. I'm not the biggest guy in the world, but I hold my own.

With any muscle, it's all about angles. You may think you're doing three exercises that are all the same, but they all are contributing in a different way. If you want to grow and do it right, you have to hit it from multiple angles. (that's what she said)

First, and foremost, the coveted bench press. It is the supreme presence in any gym. When guys are having pissing competitions, a lot of times it will lead to the bench press. The bench will test you, both mentally and physically.

You're lying on the bench, feet planted firmly on the ground, your hands are gripping the rough bar, and your back is squeezed and sturdy. You take deep breathes in and out while taking your mind to that deep, dark place. You pull the bar off the rack and now it's go-time. Just you and the bar and one of you has to lose. You slowly lower it down, controlling the dense weight as it approaches your chest. You've now reached the halfway point, shit just got real. You squeeze your elbows in and stick your chest out. Your feet are pushing against the ground as you push yourself away from the bar. It rises, oh how it rises. The glorious site of all that weight lifting back up and locking your arms. You did it. You killed it. It's almost as good as sacking a QB, but not quite.

The flat bench will definitely give you some results if you stick with it. Now as I mentioned earlier, I'm not a 3 sets of 10 kind of guy. I'm all about sets sets sets. Unless you're maxing out, which should be done MAYBE once a month, stick with more reps and sets. On my regular chest day, I will typically knock out about 10 sets ranging anywhere from 10 to 20 reps. I pyramid up and then back down.

You want to start off with a light weight. Nothing too overbearing, but enough to stretch those muscles out and get some blood pumping. Then move up in increments. I do about 25 lb increments, but everyone is different.

Once you're pushing about 75% of your max, do a couple sets. Then double up sets on each weight as you're coming back down. Doing as many as 15 sets is ok, but make sure you're listening to your body. You want to push yourself, not break yourself.

Bench Press:

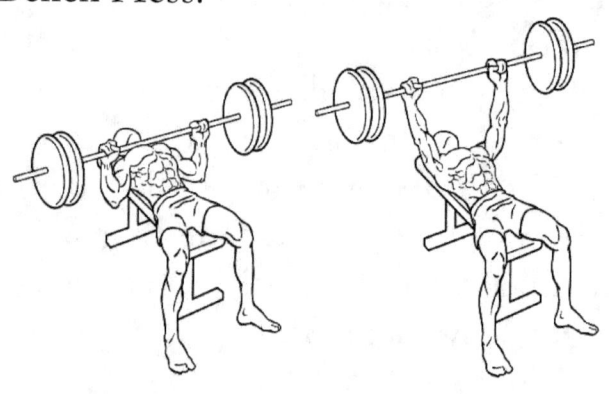

Next you want to do some sort of fly, whether it be standing cable flyes or sit down machine flyes. When it comes to chest, I like to go back and forth between pushing motions and fly motions. It gives my shoulders and tris a break between exercises.

Some people may disagree and I don't give a shit, but try not to go too heavy with flyes. After all, who the hell maxes out on flyes anyway? It puts a lot of strain on your shoulders if you don't get your angle right. Again, everyone is different, so you want to get at an angle where you feel it in your pecs. Some people like the cables higher than their shoulders, other like them to be almost even with them. Your shoulders will still get some of the pleasure, but your chest should be the main shareholder in this case.

As I said before, set and reps and reps and sets. Adjust the weight accordingly and knock out about 8 sets of 15. You want to get blood pushed into your muscles so that they grow. With any exercise, slow and steady does it. Lifting is not a race, it's an art. Make sure your feet are planted firmly on the ground and your posture is on point. No slouching and no half assed reps.

Do the same amount of sets and reps for lower cable flyes. Drop the cables all the way to the ground and grab the cold, steel handles. With this one, you want to face your palms forward and have your arms down at a 45 degree angle, slightly bent at the elbow. Slowly raise the weight and your hands should meet somewhere in the vicinity of your face. Slowly lower the weight back down and repeat.

By this point you should be catching glimpses of yourself in the magic gym mirrors and thinking, "Wow, I look pretty damn good." That's ok, we all do it, just don't be a douche bag about it. As you nonchalantly check yourself out, you make your way to the man zone.

We have arrived at the dumbbells. Find yourself a bench, recline it at a 45 degree angle, maybe a hair less, and go grab some big boy weights. Typically I will use the same weight dumbbell for an incline press, then I grab a lighter weight for a burnout set. This is just me. Listen to your body and do what best suits you.

Prop the weights on your knees, get a tight grip and pop em back. You really want to get a mind-muscle connection with this exercise and pump that chest. I am more of a power guy over looks, so I tuck my elbows in and get a nice tight press. Try to keep everything tucked and tight throughout the range of motion. If you go too far wide, it'll put a lot of pressure on your shoulder. Trust me, you don't want a jacked up rotator cup when you love lifting.

With the weights held high above you and your elbows almost locked out, slowly lower the weights down. Bring them down where it feels natural, typically around where your nips are. Lower the weights until the back of your arms are slightly lower then parallel with the deck, pause, then push em back up until they touch. Now, when you're pushing the weight back up, you want to focus on squeezing your chest. Act like you're trying to squeeze your man pecs together for a hot snapchat selfie.

Do this for about 8 sets at 12-15 reps. On the last set, grab some lighter dumbbells and push out as many as you can. Stop. I didn't say as fast as you can, I said as many as you can. Don't lose track of the basics, slow and steady. This is bodybuilding, not crossfit.

Incline Dumbbell Press:

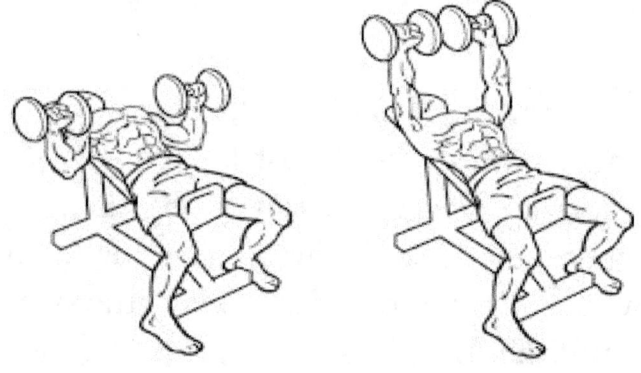

If the machine isn't already taken, make your way to the sit down fly machine. You want a good, moderate weight, nothing too crazy. Sit up straight, press your back firmly against the back, and grip the handles. With any fly, I try to leave my hands open with the handle resting in my palm. This allows you to target the chest more, as opposed to squeezing the handles and having your biceps assist. Arms slightly bent, swing in, touch your hands, and slowly release it back. Some machines have it to where you use your forearms instead of your hands. It's the same concept, just a little twist to it. Again, about 8 sets with 12-15 reps.

Machine Chest Fly (Forearm):

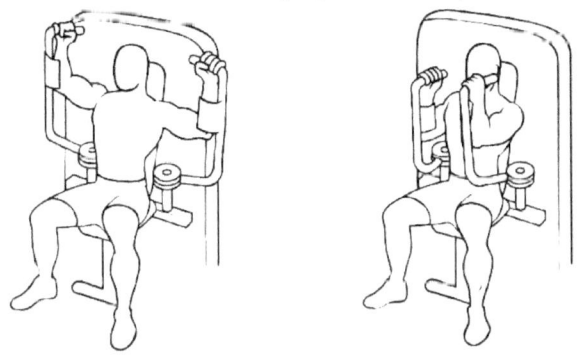

From here, there are tons of other exercises that target chest, such as the dumbbell fly, but these will get you started. You can also switch it up and do incline bench or flat dumbbell presses. Something else that I do is simple pushups. Change your hand position each set so you target different areas of your chest. Knock out about 5 sets of 30 AFTER your workout and you'll definitely feel the burn.

Dumbbell Fly:

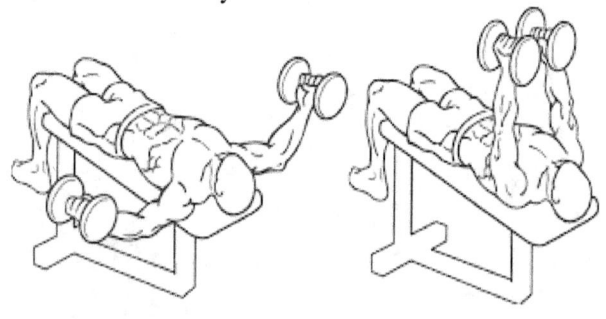

For those of you reading this and thinking, "Well, that's not how I would do it." Go play in traffic. This is a simple starter's guide for anyone that needs a little guidance. Says right there in the title, Barney Style.

CHAPTER 3

BOULDER SHOULDERS

The almighty arms. Every boy wants them, only men earn them. Now with arms, it's like a fine tuned machine. You can't have a monster engine if you don't have a tune and proper tires. Everything matters in this case and proportion is key with arms.

Sometimes I will work my shoulders in conjunction with my biceps, or sometimes I do them on back day, it all depends on how I feel. But whatever you do, make sure you warm them up first. This should go without saying, before doing any exercise, get a little warm and break a small sweat first.

Grab some 5 lb plates and hold your arms out to the side. Roll them forward and roll them backwards. Do this for a couple minutes and then we're ready to go.

We'll start with some shoulder presses. Find yourself a bench and bring the back up to almost a 90 degree angle. Slightly less to make it more comfortable. Grab a nice, medium weight and have a seat. Raise the weights next to your head with your arms at a 90 degree angle and press the weight up. Touch the dumbbells over your head and then slowly lower them back down to the original position.

The first set should really have you warmed up. Then you want to knock out another 5 or 6 sets with a medium to heavy weight. Still shoot for a 12 rep mark though. If you want, finish it off with a burnout set of a lighter weight.

Dumbbell Shoulder Press:

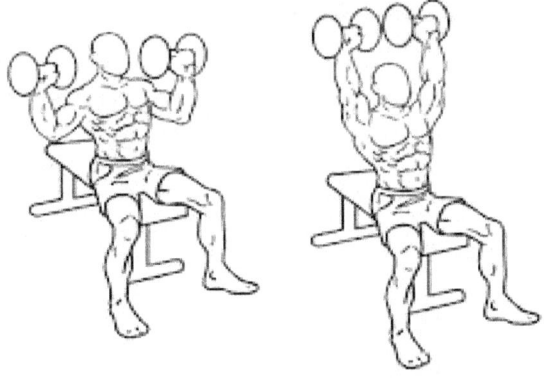

Lateral raises are one of my personal favorites. You can do these bad boys either sitting down or standing up. Usually you can't go too heavy with these. Anything from a 15 to 30 pounder will suffice, depending on your shoulders. So stand, or sit, with your arms hanging at your side, holding the weights. Face your palms in towards your body and straighten your back. Lift the weights straight out to your side until they are parallel with the deck. Then, slowly lower them back down. That's it. Easy peasy. Sounds simple, but when you're on that 4th set of 15, your shoulders start burning like chlamydia. Again, about 6 to 8 sets with high reps of about 15 to 20.

Lateral Raises:

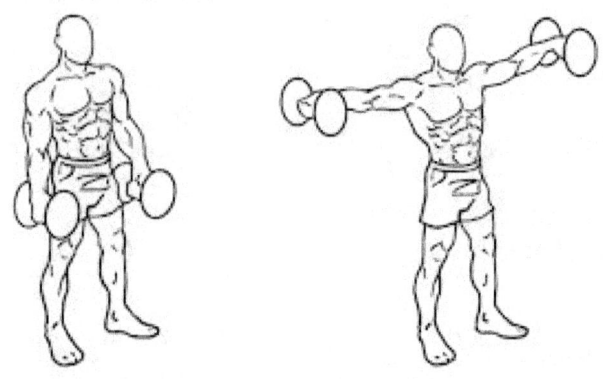

Cable raises is a good one as well. It's the same concept as above, except you do one shoulder at a time, raising your arm out and then back down. Instead of the dumbbell, you have the cable down by your feet and lift the handle outwards.

Keep in mind, angles. With these shoulder raises, cables or dumbbell, you can change the angle to hit different parts of your shoulder. You can raise them in front of you to get the front of your delt, or a 45 degree angle to hit a little bit of both.

Front Shoulder Raise:

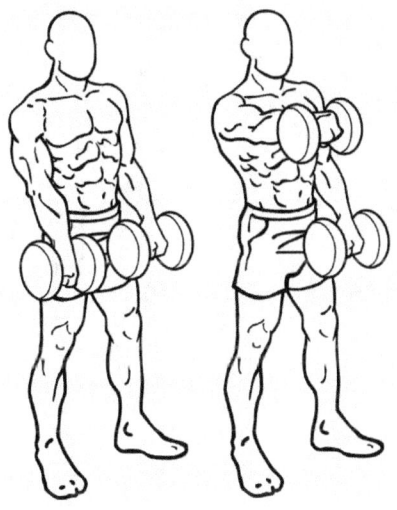

Chin raises will also target you delts and traps as well. You can do this with either a curved bar or a barbell. While standing, grab the bar with your palms facing down, a little closer than shoulder width. Start with your arms hanging straight down, then lift the bar to your chin and slowly lower it back down. Very simple movement, but targets the shoulders pretty well.

Chin Raises:

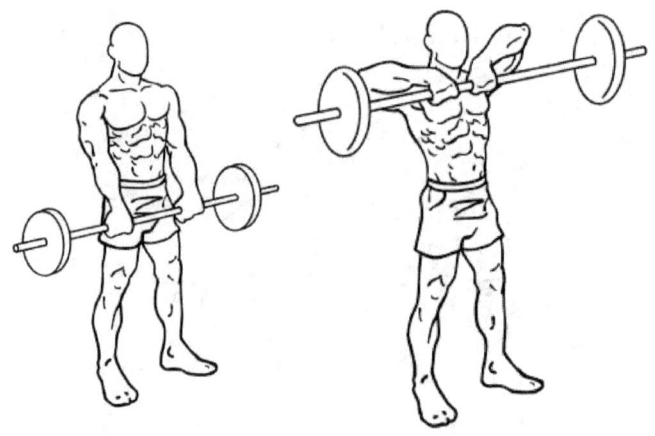

Once your shoulders start becoming more developed, you will want a more fine-tuned, well-rounded look. That is where rear delts come into play. Now there isn't a whole plethora of rear delt exercises to choose from, considering they are so small. BUT they make a huge difference in your side profile.

One simple way to hit your rear delts is to grab some very light dumbbells (10lb) and lean over at a 90 degree angle. Hang your arms down in front of you and face your palms behind you. Now raise your arms out to your side, leading with the outside of your hand. Lift until your arms are almost parallel to the ground, then slowly back down. This is a very simple and very easy exercise that targets your rear delt. A variation of this can also be done with cables.

Most of these are very simple exercises that anyone can do. Don't neglect the machines at the gym that target all the specific muscle groups as well.

CHAPTER 4

PONY KICKED

Triceps, the foundation of big arms. Without them, you have small arms. Sorry bros, it's a harsh truth.

You ever see someone with biceps an no triceps? Kind of looks like a stick with a cyst on it? Then you see a guy with triceps and nothing else, he still looks kind of big. Triceps are something that everyone should put on their priority list. Nothing is better than flexing the back of your arm and it looks like a unicorn stomped you in it. We all want the horseshoe.

One of the most popular tri exercises is the rope pull down. Simply put, there is a rope, you grab it, and pull it down. The rope should be dangling right in front of your face....lol. Grab each end with your hands and pin your elbows to your side. Your arms should be at a 90 degree angle pointing in front of you. Now with only bending your elbows, pull the rope down and then kick em out to the side. Flex your triceps and squeeze when you kick em out. You want to push blood into your muscle and make em grow!!

Rope Pull Down:

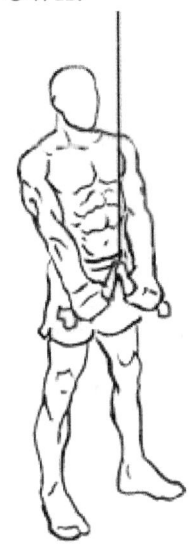

There is a variation that can also be done with a straight bar. In this case, you would face your palms down and pin your elbows to your side. Push down, straighten your arms out and flex! Then a slow release back up. The rope will target the outside head of the tricep and the straight bar will get the short head, towards the back of your arm. I can't stress enough how important the negative rep is with any exercise. Slow flex, slow release.

Standing tricep extensions. This is also used with the rope, except this time it's behind you. Put the cable lower than your shoulders. Some people put it close to the ground, others put it about mid-back. It's your choice. To start, grab the rope behind you and have your elbows bent with your hands above your shoulders. Extend your arms up and forward, like you're throwing a soccer ball with 2 hands from behind your head.

Standing Tricep Extensions:

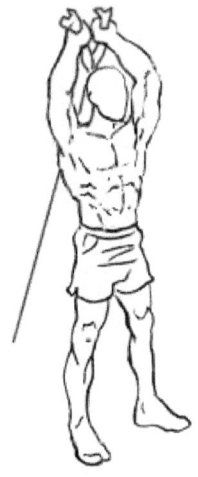

Cables give you a smooth range of motion when it comes to any sort of tricep extension, but we can't neglect the dumbbells. One exercise that you might see often is the sitting dumbbell tricep extension. This only requires one dumbbell, but both hands.

Sit down with your back straight and your chest out. Grab a fairly heavy dumbbell and stand it up. Next, you want to lift it under the top end and raise it over your head. Bending at the elbow, slowly lower it bchind your head and the lift it back up. Simple stuff.

Dumbbell Tricep Extension:

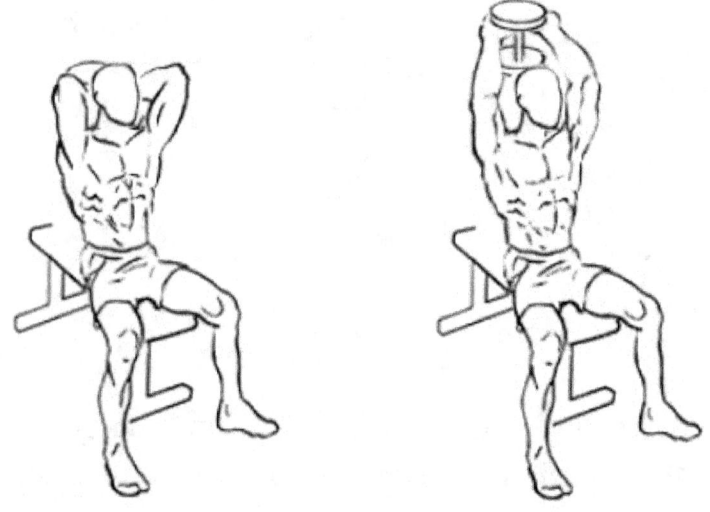

Another dumbbell variation for the triceps is the dumbbell kickback. Now with this one, you only do one arm at a time. Starting with the left, because we always start with the left oorah, place your right hand and right knee flat on the bench,. Your left leg is standing off to the side and your left hand is holding the dumbbell. Sounds difficult, luckily I have pictures. Pin your left elbow to your side and bend your arm to a 90 degree angle. Now kick that monkey back. Extend your elbow and push the dumbbell backwards towards your ass. Flex and squeeze, then slowly bring it back down. As promised, here is the picture....

Dumbbell Tricep Kickbacks:

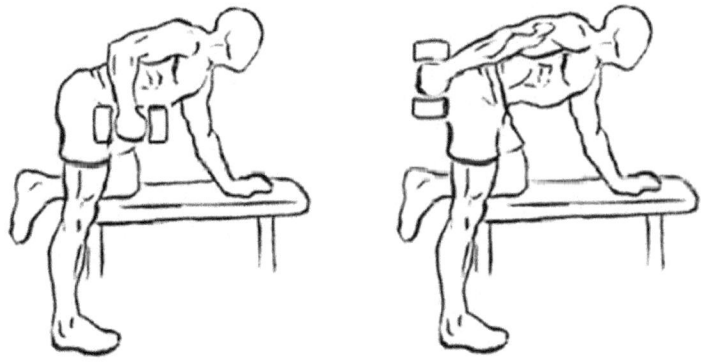

Dips are one of my favorites. They really work your triceps and target some of your chest as well. These can be done on a machine or by using a bench. Some machines have weights to assist if you are still building up your strength. But for the most part, you hold yourself up with the 2 bars provided. With your body hanging in the air, lower yourself down until your arms reach a 90 degree angle, then push yourself back up to the starting position. I usually like to knock out around 5 to 8 sets of these. They really burn your tris up pretty quick.

Dips:

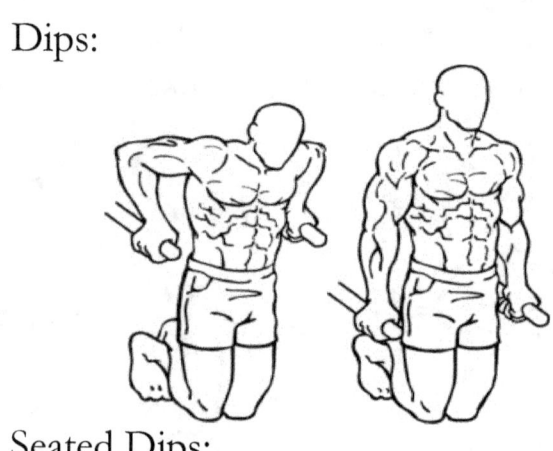

Seated Dips:

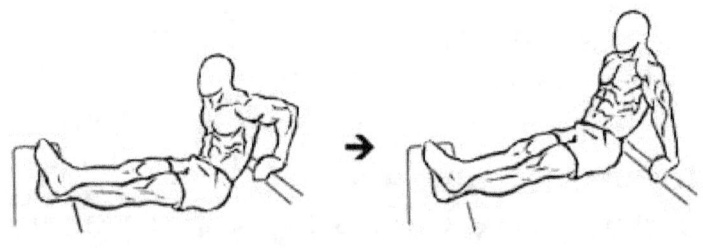

Again, there are plenty of other tricep exercises, such as the single arm cable extension, but these should be enough to give you a pretty sweet workout. With triceps, I like em to burn, so you want to do about 10 sets with high reps. We're talking 20 to 30 reps on each set.

CHAPTER 5

APPLE SLEEVES

Biceps have always been one of the trademark muscles for bodybuilders. From the 70s to now, you will always see guys posing and flexing their biceps. Curls get the girls. Let's be honest, when you have a nice rounded bicep, it looks pretty damn good stacked with some big shoulders and tris.

Curls will always be one of the best exercises to build bulging biceps. All other exercises are just different variations of the curl. You know why? Because angles, that's why. Hit that shit from every angle you can. A curl is simple, but a good curl is mental. While standing, or sitting, grab 2 dumbbells and hold one in each hand. While alternating arms, try to face your palm up and curl the dumbbell up, as if you are trying to touch it to your shoulder.

SLOWLY lower it back down and do the same with the other arm.

Now I say it's mental. A lot of this is because the movement itself is a very simple movement. However, it's very easy for one just to curl the weight up and down carelessly. You want to really focus on that curl and squeeze as you curl it. Flex so hard your bicep feels like it's going to explode. You want to concentrate on it like you are trying to master this simple movement. Don't even think about curling with your other arm until your first one is down and you are ready to give your undivided attention to it.

You will want to do as many sets and reps as you can. The more the better. Torture your biceps and make them burn, because that is the only way that they will grow into apples under your skin,

Dumbbell Bicep Curl:

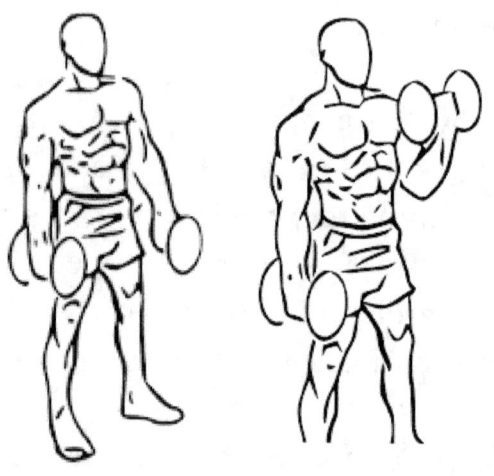

Now, I hope you're ready to repent your sins, because we're moving on to the preacher curls. This is the same movement, for the most part, except this is a lot more concentrated and will really flex those biceps. I'll go over the seated preacher curls and then we'll touch on the standing one arm.

While sitting at the holy preacher curl bench, grab yourself a nice weighted ez bar and say your prayers. You want to grab the bar and face your palms up. Scoot all the way forward so that the pad is pushed up against your chest and in your armpits. Those big tris should be flat against the pad and arms bent, holding the bar up. Slowly lower it down and fight the weight with those little biceps. Don't let the bar win, Lower it all the way down, then pull that sum'bitch back up.

These will really test you and THAT'S what we want to do. We don't want any bitch weight. We want to work those damn muscles and tear em up.

Seated Preacher Curls:

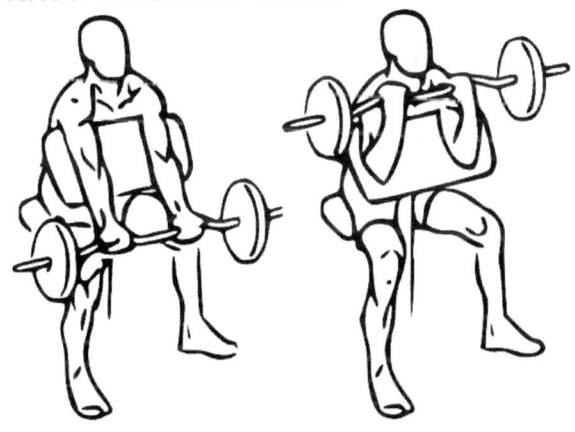

Standing Dumbbell Preacher Curls:

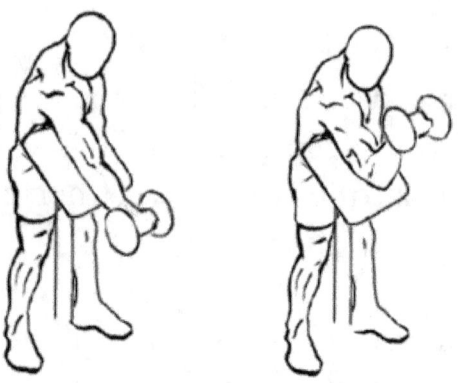

A more concentrated dumbbell curl is to sit down and do one arm at a time. Grab your dumbbell and hold it in between your legs. Rest your elbow on the inside of your knee and curl the weight up. This allows you to just use your bicep and not have any other muscles assist in the lift.

Seated Dumbbell Curl:

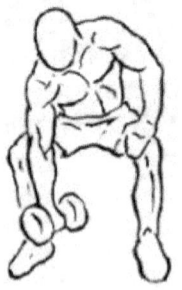 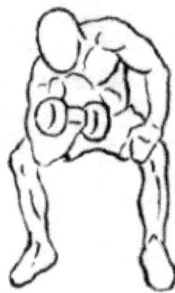

A nice way I like to end my bicep workout is to crank out some curls with the ez bar. I just do set after set until I can't lift my arms anymore. This really pumps blood into the muscle and forces them to grow.

Standing up, grab the ez bar and pin your elbows to your sides. Squeeze and curl that bad boy up and then back down. Do this as many times as you can.

EZ Bar Curl:

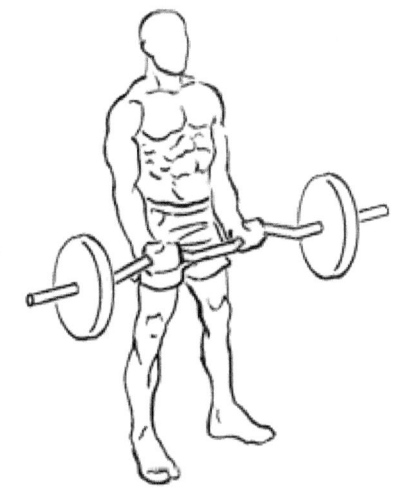

CHAPTER 6

SPREAD YOUR WINGS

One thing that people sometimes neglect, aside from legs, is their back. Too often they get caught up with wanting to have a big chest and sleeve-ripping guns. Well, let me let you in on a little secret, chicks love ripped backs.

In order to spread our wings, we need to build up some giant lats. One of the most obvious exercises for that is the lat pulldown. This is a seated machine with bar hanging above you. You want to grab the bar wide and keep your back straight. Now pull the bar down and towards your chest. The thing is, your muscles grow the way you train them, so you want to get a wide grip on the bar so that you can grow some wide lats.

You can also do this with a close grip handle. Same concept. Sit up, grab the handles and pull down and inwards to your chest. This particular exercise will also work your lats, but since your elbows are closer to your body, this will also work the rhomboids between your shoulder blades of glory.

With both of these exercises, it's easy to use your arms too much and get your biceps tired out. It's a mental thing, but try to pull and squeeze with your back, as opposed to just pulling with your arms. You're going to want to do about 8 sets at 15 reps.

Lat Pull:

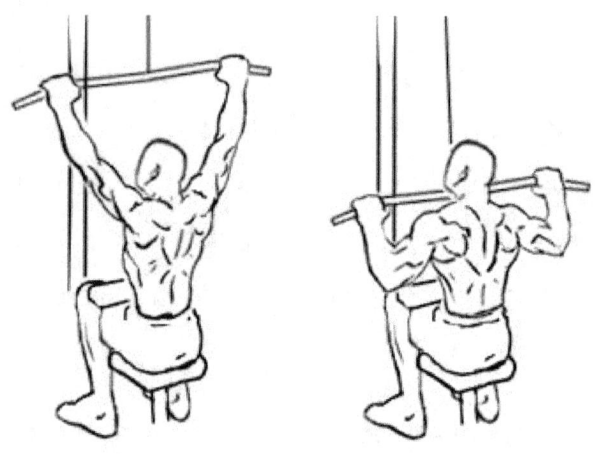

Another back exercise that I have grown to love is the seated row. This can also be done with a long, wide handle, but it's typically done with the close grip.

You're going to place your feet in front of you, on the plate that is for your feet, Crazy how that works, right? Sit up straight and grab the handle. Your arms will be sticking straight in front of you. Now slightly lean back, not a lot, and pull your arms back. You want to keep your elbows close to your body as you're pulling back. Again, remember to pull and squeeze with your back, instead of simply pulling the weight with your arms.

Seated Rows:

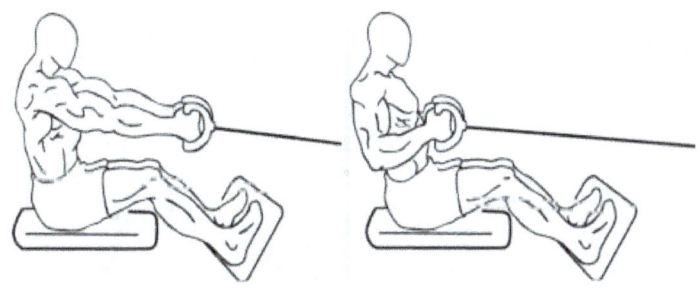

We can't forget about the dumbbells. Don't get me wrong, machines are great, but something about dumbbells is so primitive and really gives you a nice pump.

For back, we'll start our dumbbell fiasco with some chainsaws. There are other, more technical, names out there, but chainsaws just sounds bad ass. This one is similar to the tricep kickbacks I mentioned earlier (pg. 31). Get a bench and put your right hand and right knee on the bench. With the dumbbell hanging in your left hand, pull your elbow back towards your hip like you're trying to start a chainsaw. Knock out about 15, then switch hands.

Chainsaws:

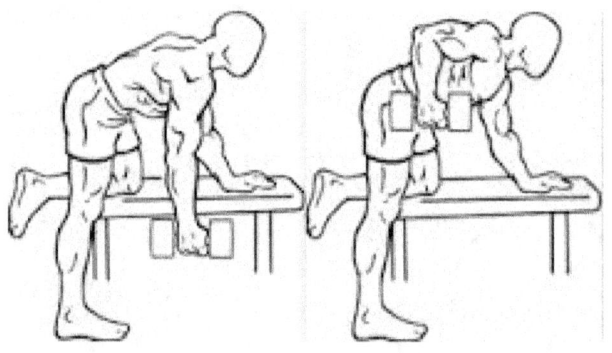

Also with the dumbbells, we got the reverse fly. This is done by lying face down on a flat bench. You want to make sure the bench is tall enough, because your arms will be hanging in front of you. Putting the bench at a slight incline will also work. So, now that you're face down with your arms hanging, lift your arms outwards like your spreading your arms to fly. Keep your palms facing the ground and slowly lower it back down. Remember to squeeze with your back as you do this.

Reverse Fly:

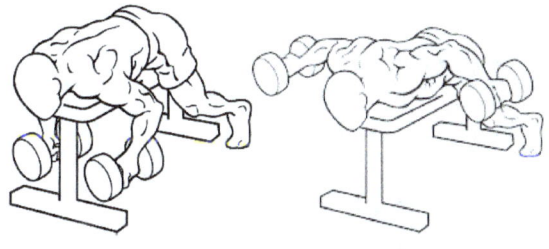

After dumbbells, come barbells. You can't neglect the backbone of the weight room. Nothing like the sound of iron clanging together in a room full of sweaty dudes….wait….

This one can feel awkward at first, but once you get your posture right, you'll see the wonders of its glory. We're talking about barbell rows. You start out with the bar on the ground in front of you, and both your feet at shoulder's width apart. Grab the bar with an underhand grip and straighten out your back. (An overhand grip can also be utilized.) You want to lean over, but not slouch your back in the process. Now pull the bar towards your stomach and lower it back down.

Barbell Rows:

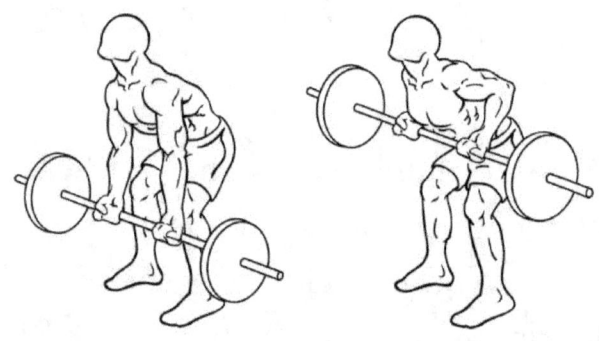

A variety of back exercises can also be done by utilizing the cables and other machines provided by your happy, friendly neighborhood gym.

CHAPTER 7

TREE TRUNKS

Leg day, everyone wants to skip it. Well, weak bitches. Working out your legs is paramount for the rest of your body to grow. It is such a large muscle group that it will boost some testosterone and kick up that metabolism to help burn some fat.

Since we just covered back, I'm going to start with deadlifts. I say this because it easily falls under both back and legs. Deadlifts are one of the most important exercises for building, strength, mass, power, and core. It's just the way it is folks. If you're not doing deadlifts, start doing that shit.

With anything, form is just as important as condoms on prom night. Start off with a light weight until you get your form correct and build some strength.

Start off standing in front of the bar with your feet shoulder width apart. You want your feet to be about midway under it. Bend at your waist and grab the bar about shoulder width. You can either do a double overhand grip, or one over and one under. If the weight isn't that heavy, then a double over will suffice.

Next, bend at your knees and drop down until your shins touch the bar. Be sure not to roll the bar while doing this. Then stick your chest out and straighten your back. You want to keep a straight back during this whole exercise. Now take a deep breath and push up with your legs while keeping the bar close to your body. You want to tighten your core during this movement. Pull your shoulders back, lock your legs, and squeeze your ass at the top. Then slowly lower it back down.

Deadlift:

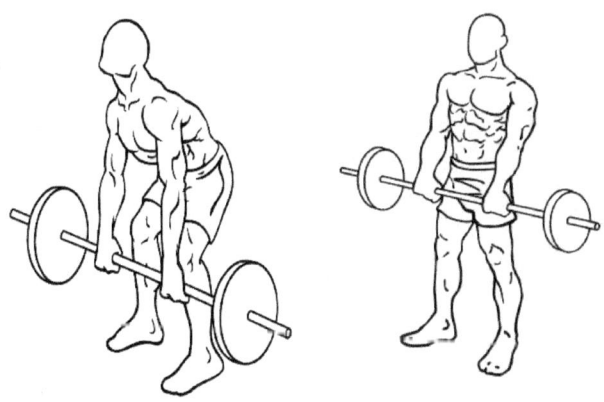

The number one exercise for building some strong, stout tree trunk legs....squats. It would even be ok if you knocked out some squats every day. Hell, sometimes I knock out a couple sets of squats on chest day so I can get my blood and testosterone pumping.

Good form and a firm foundation are necessary for squats. You might want to have some music to pump you up too.

Step up to the bar and grab it firmly with both hands. You want to have your hands about shoulder width apart. Duck your head under the bar and place it on those pads we call traps. Next, plant your feet about shoulder width apart, maybe a little wider. Lift the weight up and take a small step back from the rack. Now the fun is beginning. Take a deep breath and hold it in your stomach. While keeping your back straight, bend your legs and push your ass back. We're going low, ass to the grass. Drop it like it's hot all the way down then explode up and thrust your hips forward.

Squat:

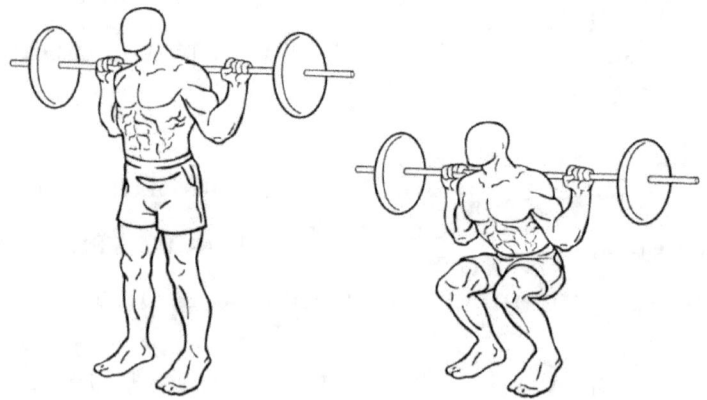

Using a belt is highly advised for safety purposes. A lot of people tend to want to lean over while doing a squat. No. Negative. Get that shit outta here. It's all in the hips and pushing from the heels of your feet. Push your ass back like an Instagram thot, then thrust your hips forward like you're trying to spread your family name.

Maxing out on squats will tell the true strength of a man, just like bench and deadlifts do. So unless you're maxing out, I like to do about 10 to 12 sets of squats. A nice 75% of your max at about 12 to 15 reps.

One of my favorites is the front squat. This is almost the same as a squat, except you hold the bar in front of you, resting on your shoulders. This really works your core as well as your legs.

Front Squat:

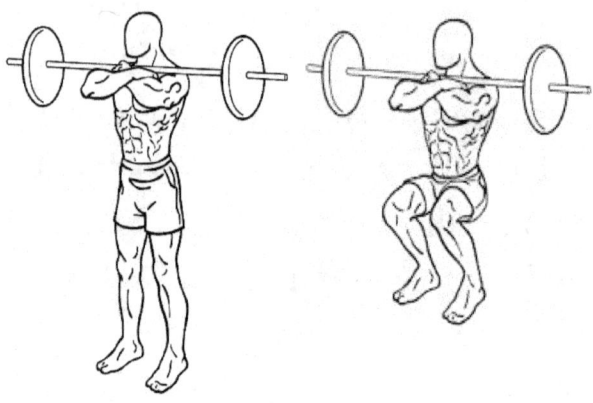

So now we move on to the machines. First is the leg extension. This works your quads so you get a nice tear drop in those tree trunks.

With this machine, you sit down and adjust it to your leg length. The bar that is being lifted should sit a tad higher than your ankles. Grab the handles to your side and kick your feet up, straightening your legs, then slowly lower it back down. A nice medium weight is good for these as it puts a little stress on your knees. Knock out about 8 sets at 12 to 15 reps.

Leg Extensions:

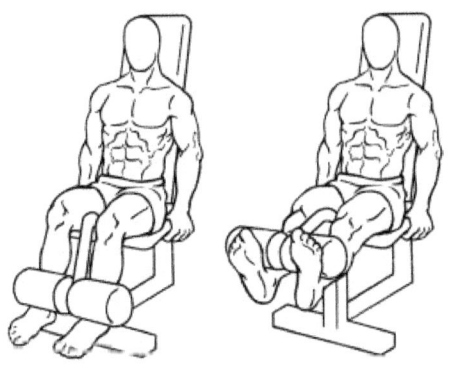

Leg curls target your hammy on the back of your legs. It's like the bicep of your leg. There are a few variations of the leg curl machine, but we're talking about the face down one.

Lay face down on the machine and place the bar on your calves, maybe a hair lower. Grip the handles to brace yourself, then bend your knees and curl your legs like your trying to touch them to your ass. Slowly lower it back down and you've done it. 8 sets, 12-15 reps.

Leg Curls:

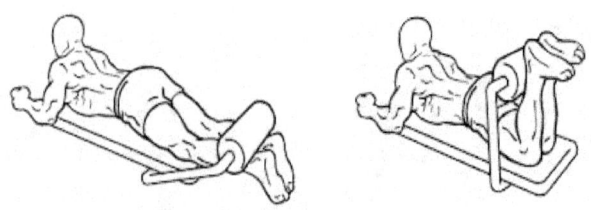

The last leg exercise we'll cover is the leg press. This is another power movement like the squat. Simply put, load the plates, place your feet about shoulder width apart, bring your knees to your chest then explode from your heels.

Leg Press:

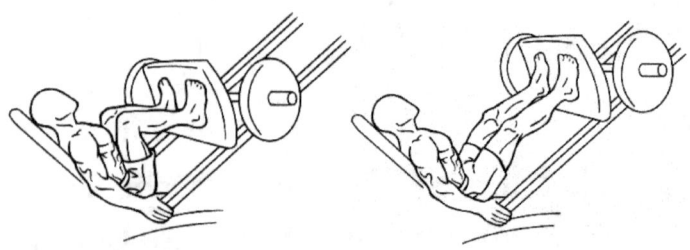

These 5 or 6 exercises are plenty to get you through a full leg day. About 8 to 10 sets of each at about 15 reps. You'll definitely have some issues getting out of bed and sitting on the toilet. Gonna look like a baby deer the next couple days.

For those of you asking about calves, just do calf raises ever chance you get. Calves are genetic, but luckily can be built. Fortunately, I was blessed with calves, so I'm not sure what to tell you on this one. Sorry...

CHAPTER 8

THE BIG THREE

The holy trinity of putting on mass, size and gaining power is:

Squat – Bench – Deadlift.

These 3 power movements are the supreme exercises for any powerlifter, football player, meathead, bouncer, and any other big ass dude who's big as shit. This is the core of building a strong body. These 3 really measure a man because they are compound movements and test total body strength.

If you were to throw away everything that you have read so far and only did these three exercises, you would still see some pretty significant gains. Remember when I talked about "thinking big"? This is what I was referring to. This is that old school, raw, uncut, unfiltered, don't give a shit power.

The bench press obviously works the pecs, which is a good sized muscle. This gives you a stout upper body and gives you great power when it comes to pushing motions.

Squats work your legs which is a HUGE muscle group. It gets your hams, glutes, quads, hit some core, all that goodness. So now you have a nice foundation to carry that huge chest around.

Then the deadlifts. One of the most beneficial exercises for targeting multiple backs muscles, leg muscles, and hitting your core. Your core is important because it works your pelvis, lower back, hips and abdomen. This leads to better balance and stability. So this is especially beneficial for athletes.

Now you have solid body with a strong core, strong back, sturdy legs, and a menacing chest. So whatever you decide to do with your workout plans, make sure that these 3 are somehow incorporated into it.

If you are in one of those moods to stay at the gym for a few hours and get a kick ass workout, do the big 3 on the same day. Start off with some squats and knock out about 12 sets. Don't go crazy heavy, that's the thing. Keep everything in moderation. Throw on about 225 and knock our 12 sets of 12 or 15. Obviously it will be different for everyone, but a nice medium weight so that you can knock out high reps and sets.

From here, you can either let your legs rest and go to bench, or jump right into deadlifts. I would personally go to bench so I would have fresh legs for the deadlifts.

So on bench, same thing, about 12 sets of a good medium weight. Shoot for a 15 rep target and knock out as many as you can. On the last couple sets, just throw on one plate and do some burnouts. That light weight will feel like 1,000 lbs after you've done 10 sets though.

Then the deadlifts. Take you a short water break then get right into it. By this point your body should be plenty warmed up and you might even feel nauseous. Good, cuz if you ain't dyin' then you ain't tryin'. Same thing here, medium weight and knock out as many as you can. 10 to 12 sets for about 12 reps.

If you can manage to do this, you will have one of the best, most glorifying, muscle pumping work outs of your life. You'll leave the gym feeling like a Viking.

CHAPTER 9

DIET. . . UGH

Diet, just saying it makes me hungry. Now I'm not going to get on here and tell you about fasting and counting macros and all that other bullshit that people feed to you. Straight up, you want to get big, you got to eat big.

This is going to be a realistic meal plan that you can incorporate into your life. It's not even a meal plan, it's just shit that I eat.

Without further ado, the proteins. This is the foundation of my diet. I don't care what else I do or don't eat, the main concern is making sure that I am getting my protein. I'm simple when it comes to mine and eat plenty of it. This is what helps you grow. This is what makes all that time put in at the gym worth it. You're constantly breaking your muscles down and ripping those fibers up. Consuming protein helps heal and rebuild those muscles.

In no particular order, these are my main sources of protein: Chicken breast, turkey, tuna, other fish, red meat, black beans, quinoa. Ok well, that was pretty much the order from most consumed to least, but I do eat a lot of black beans.

For fruit and veggies, try to go fresh with it. Nothing is better than some fresh produce. Anything green is typically good. Broccoli, green beans, carrots, bananas, etc. etc. I don't care what kind you eat, just make sure that you eat PLENTY of them. Fruit is good, but they do have sugars. It's not the same kind of sugar as soda and candy, but just make sure your main focus is veggies. Veggies are full of all sorts of vitamins and nutrients that are essential for getting and keeping a healthy body. Juicing is always an option as well. Now, I don't mean go on an all-juice diet, I just mean incorporate it into your diet so that you get your fair share of fruits and veggies.

Carbs, damn I love carbs. They are the glue that holds the world together, but we have to be careful not to indulge too much. I'm not going to sit here and tell you that I don't eat carbs, because I do, and that's ok. Carbs are fuel for our bodies. So if you play sports or run marathons, (who would run a marathon??) you may carb load in order to have fuel. But if you consume mass amounts of carbs and don't burn them off, they get stored in your body and you get fat.

The time that you eat carbs can matter. If you have some for breakfast or lunch, that's ok. You're going to be up and active throughout the day so you will use and burn them. Having them with a late dinner, not so much. Your body goes into shutdown mode when you go to bed and you won't burn as many carbs as you would throughout the day. So just be mindful of how many and when you decide to eat your carbs.

Sweets. Don't eat them. It's easy for me to say because I don't have a huge sweet-tooth. I have something sweet maybe once or twice a week. But please please please don't make a meal out of a box of honeybuns.

How often should you eat? Well, for me, I eat my three big meals a day and I eat smaller meals/snacks in between. So you could say about 5 times a day. A quick example would be: 5 eggs for breakfast, protein bar, then 2 cans of tuna for lunch, small turkey sandwich, then a large chicken breast with veggies for dinner. That is a regular day for me. Some people do 6 to 8 meals a day. Like I mentioned earlier, if you want to get big, you have to eat big.

Supplements are great, they do exactly that, supplement. Having protein shakes a few times a day can help someone who may not have a big appetite for food. I know lots of people who take 8 different types of supplements. As for me, I keep it simple. I like to do a pre-workout, some BCAAs, and protein. My main source of vitamins, nutrients, and protein is from my food. Food is the best supplement that you can put into your body.

So long story short, eat plenty of food, real food, good food, not junk food. A quick rule of thumb at the grocery store is to do all your shopping on the perimeter. Produce, meat, dairy, eggs, everything is on the perimeter. All that stuff in the middle is junk.....usually.

CHAPTER 10

REAL TALK

All jokes aside, let me get on some real shit to end this thing. Some of you get on this bodybuilding train because you or your friends get on a little kick or because it's the fad thing to do. Scratch that shit. If you want this, it's a way of life. For those that love it, you eat-sleep-lift. You don't post about it on Facebook or the Gram, that's because it's nothing significant. It's not a special event or something new. Training your body is something as normal as breathing to us.

Once you decide that you want to make this part of your life, don't let anything stand in your way. Let's be real with ourselves, you only need about an hour or an hour and a half to get a good workout in. The only bar you should be concerned with is the barbell. Put your phone on silent, shut down Facebook, tell everyone you'll be back in an hour.

The only one that can get in the way of your dream is you. There are so many examples of people who went through life with the cards stacked against them and STILL crushed their goals and accomplished their dreams. There are no excuses to not reach the goals that you have set for yourself.

I once told myself that I wouldn't be able to write a book because I worked too much and had too much going on. Well, here I am on the last chapter of this book and I'm also writing another book. It CAN be done, it's just a matter of how bad you want it. I don't care where you grew up, what conditions you live in, your bad circumstances, anything.

If you want something bad enough then you need to pick your ass up and go out there and take it. No one is going to give you handouts throughout your life and that's especially true with working out. If you slack, the results will show. You have to earn every bit of this.

What is talent if it's not utilized? What is hard work if it's not applied? Don't waste the opportunity to leave your legacy behind. Do not waste the chance to leave your mark in this world. You can have all the talent and tools in the world, but it all means nothing without effort. Effort separates the ones who really want it and the ones who settle with what they have. You have to get out there and take it. No one is going to rep your sets, score your points, or make your tackles. Only you can do that for yourself. Go out there and seize the day or die regretting all the time you've lost.